EASY FITNESS EXERCISE FOR SENIORS TO LOSE WEIGHT

The Complete Beginners Guide to Enhance Flexibility, Improve Core strength and Balance 6 minutes Daily

Anthony C. Welborn

Copyright © 2024 Anthony C. Welborn

All rights reserved. No portion of this publication may be reproduced, distributed,or transmitted in any form of by any means, including photocopying, recording,or other electronic or mechanical methods, without the prior writing permission of the publisher, except in the case of brief quotations embodied in critical reviews and certain Copyrightothers noncommercial uses permitted by copyright

TABLE OF CONTENT

INTRODUCTION.. **6**
CHAPTER ONE.. **13**
   Basic Anatomy and Physiology............................*13*
   Safety Guidelines for Seniors...............................*17*
   Setting Realistic Fitness Goals............................ *22*
   Creating a Supportive Exercise Environment........*25*
CHAPTER TWO.. **31**
   Flexibility Training for Seniors............................ *31*
   Benefits of Flexibility Exercises............................*35*
   Upper Body Stretching Techniques....................... *38*
   Lower Body Stretching Techniques....................... *42*
   Core Flexibility Exercises.................................... *46*
   Integrated Flexibility Routine............................*49*
CHAPTER THREE..**55**
   Core Strength Exercises for Seniors.......................*55*
   Importance of Core Strength for Seniors................*57*
   Core Activation Techniques..................................*62*
   Abdominal Strengthening Exercises......................*65*
   Back Strengthening Exercises..............................*70*
   Total Core Strength Workout Routine....................*74*
CHAPTER FOUR..**79**
   Balance and Stability Training..............................*79*
   Static Balance Exercises....................................... *87*
   Dynamic Balance Exercises................................... *91*
   Proprioception Training.. *94*

  Complete Balance Workout Plan............................ 100
 CHAPTER FIVE...105
  Sample Workouts for Seniors................................105
  Beginner's Workout Routine................................ 108
  Intermediate Exercise Plan.................................... 111
  Advanced Fitness Program....................................115
  Chair-Based Workout Options..............................118
  Quick and Efficient Exercise Routines................... 122
 CHAPTER SIX...126
  Nutrition Tips for Seniors.. 127
  Importance of Nutrition for Older Adults.............. 131
  Balanced Meal Planning for Weight Loss..............135
  Nutrient-Rich Foods for Seniors............................ 138
  Healthy Snacking Strategies...................................141
  Lifestyle Factors for Healthy Aging......................146
 CONCLUSION...149

INTRODUCTION

In the vast metropolis of New Fountain, amidst the towering skyscrapers and the constant rush and bustle of metropolitan life, lives a lady named Mariam. Mariam, who is in her late fifties, exudes a serene elegance and an unwavering energy that defies her age. Her life has been full of victories and struggles, but she has stayed strong and determined to live it to the fullest.

Despite her apparent strength, Mariam has been quietly dealing with the consequences of a sedentary lifestyle she had unknowingly acquired in the past. As a corporate executive, Mariam noticed the gradual emergence of symptoms around her waist, wrists, and ankles after sitting for lengthy periods at her desk. At first, she ignored these discomforts as minor inconveniences, attributing them to the stress of her busy profession. However, as time went on, the symptoms became greater, accompanied by a constant sensation of weakness that appeared to sap her energies.

Mariam found herself at a crossroads after becoming aware of the health risks associated with her sedentary lifestyle. She knew that if she stayed on this road, her quality of life would worsen, and she would face more significant health difficulties in the future.

It was a sobering reality that motivated Mariam to take action and find a way to recover her health and vigor.

In her search for answers, Mariam came upon this book that proved to transform her attitude to well-being. Intrigued by the prospect of finding a solution to her problems, she enthusiastically dug into its pages, soaking up its knowledge and executing its advice with steadfast devotion.

This book acted as a road map to healthy living, taking Mariam on the rightful path of self-discovery and empowerment. It underlined the need to include regular physical activity in her daily routine, recommending basic yet effective workouts that could be readily included in her hectic schedule.

Mariam gladly accepted these ideas, progressively introducing more activity into her life and breaking free from the constraints of her sedentary lifestyle. She began going for brief walks during her lunch breaks, doing light stretching exercises in the morning, and even experimenting with yoga and tai chi to strengthen her body and relax her mind.

As Mariam began to focus on her health and well-being, she saw an amazing change inside herself. The aches that had previously plagued her everyday life began to fade, replaced with a renewed sense of vibrancy and energy. She started feeling much better, energetic and healthy.

Perhaps the most significant alteration of all was Mariam's newfound sense of empowerment, which pervaded every part of her existence. No longer limited by her history, she saw each day as a chance to grow, explore, and appreciate the gift of health that she had regained through her resolve and effort.

In the end, Mariam's story demonstrates the transformational potential of self-care and perseverance. Her unrelenting dedication to prioritizing her health not only restored control over her physical well-being but also unlocked a renewed feeling of vibrancy and purpose, illuminating her way forward.

As she embraces each new day with renewed vigor and thankfulness, Mariam serves as a light of encouragement for everyone who dares to begin on their path to recovery and fulfillment.

I Celebrate Progress Small or Big on My fitness Path

CHAPTER ONE

Basic Anatomy and Physiology

Swimming or water aerobics is a fantastic activity for seniors looking to reduce weight. These exercises give a full-body workout while putting less strain on the joints. The buoyancy of water decreases the danger of damage while yet allowing for range-of-motion workouts.

Tai chi is another great kind of exercise. This ancient Chinese martial art emphasizes slow, flowing motions that enhance balance, flexibility, and strength. Tai chi is easy on the joints and may be adjusted to suit different fitness levels.

Yoga is also beneficial for elders since it improves flexibility, balance, and strength via a variety of poses and stretches. Yoga also promotes relaxation and stress reduction, which improves both physical and mental health.

Walking is a great option for elders. Brisk walking has cardiovascular advantages and may be readily included in regular activities. It's low-impact and can be tailored to different fitness levels.

Strength training routines with modest weights or resistance bands are particularly important for seniors in maintaining muscle mass and bone density. Concentrate on activities that work key muscular groups, such as squats, lunges, and bicep curls.

To avoid injury, always warm up before you exercise and cool down afterward.

Listen to your body and adjust the workouts as required. Before beginning any new fitness regimen, speak with a healthcare expert, especially if you have pre-existing health concerns.

Consistency is essential for seeing results, so try including a variety of workouts in your program and get the advantages of increased fitness and general well-being.

Safety Guidelines for Seniors

When engaging in workout routines aimed at weight reduction, it is essential to consider safety to avoid accidents and enhance overall wellness.

Before beginning any fitness program, seniors should contact their healthcare physician to verify they are healthy enough to engage in physical exercise. This stage aids in the identification of any possible dangers or restrictions unique to the individual.

Start Slowly and Progress Seniors should start with low-impact exercises like walking, swimming, or cycling, then gradually increase the intensity and duration as their strength and endurance improve. This strategy reduces the chance of strain or damage.

Proper Warm-up and Cool-down: Before exercising, seniors should warm up gently to prepare their muscles and joints for action. Fainting and dizziness is prevented and heart rate is reduced through cool down time.

Focus on Balance and Stability: Including activities that improve balance and stability, such as yoga or tai chi, lowers the chance of falling, which is a common worry for seniors.

Use of Proper Equipment: Make sure elders have access to suitable footwear and apparel for their chosen activities to avoid slips, trips, and falls. Consider utilizing supporting equipment, such as walking poles or resistance bands, to help you exercise safely.

Stay Hydrated: Proper hydration is critical throughout the exercise to avoid dehydration and maintain peak performance. Encourage elders to consume water before, during, and after exercise.

Listen to Your Body: Seniors should monitor how their bodies feel during exercise and modify the intensity or length accordingly. Encourage them to stop if they feel any discomfort, dizziness, or shortness of breath. Monitoring and evaluation should be done regularly to ensure that the fitness program remains safe and effective.

Following these safety precautions allows seniors to confidently begin on a fitness path focused on weight loss while reducing the chance of injury or setbacks. When it comes to encouraging health and well-being in older individuals, always prioritize safety.

Setting Realistic Fitness Goals

Setting realistic training goals is particularly crucial for seniors who wish to lose weight. Begin by assessing your current fitness level, taking into account age, health concerns, and mobility. Consult a healthcare provider or fitness professional to ensure safety and suitability.

When setting goals, look for ones that are feasible and suitable to your abilities and lifestyle. Consider both short-term and long-term objectives, such as increasing regular activity, improving flexibility, or losing a specified amount of weight over a reasonable time frame.

Prioritize consistency above intensity. Slowly include modest physical routines into your everyday routine, such as walking, swimming, or moderate stretching. Aim for at least 150 minutes of moderate aerobic exercise each week, supplemented with strength training activities focusing on major muscle groups twice per week.

Take note of your body's signals and adjust your goals accordingly. Listen for any discomfort or pain and modify your activity to avoid injury. Stay hydrated and consume nutritious meals to support your fitness journey.

Regularly recording your progress can help you stay motivated and accountable. To stay on track, keep an activity record, use fitness apps, or ask a workout buddy or coach for help.

Celebrate little victories along the way, and be patient with yourself. Understand that your progress may be slower than that of younger individuals, but perseverance and patience will pay off in the end.

The key to successful weight loss and overall fitness is to develop long-term habits and make gradual lifestyle changes. Setting sensible goals and adhering to a balanced approach will help you retain good health and well-being far into your retirement years.

Creating a Supportive Exercise Environment

Creating a supportive workout environment for elders looking to reduce weight requires many critical aspects. First, make sure the room is secure and accessible, free of clutter and risks. Arrange equipment in an orderly fashion to aid navigation. In addition, provide enough lighting and ventilation to improve comfort and safety during workouts.

Encourage social interaction by creating an inviting environment. Set up group training sessions or partner exercises to foster friendship and motivation. Include music playlists with upbeat songs to improve the entire experience and promote exercise.

Offer a choice of exercise activities customized to elders' needs and abilities. Include low-impact activities like walking, swimming, or chair exercises to suit those with varying fitness levels and mobility constraints. Offer flexibility exercises to enhance range of motion and minimize stiffness, as well as strength training to increase muscle growth and metabolism.

Ensure sufficient education and supervision to avoid injuries and maintain proper form. Hire competent fitness instructors who have worked with elders and can give direction and assistance. Provide tailored care and changes as needed to address unique health problems or physical constraints.

Create a positive reinforcement system to acknowledge accomplishments and growth. Implement prizes or acknowledgments for meeting goals and adhering to workout programs. Encourage self-monitoring and goal-setting to help elders take control of their fitness journey.

Create a friendly communal atmosphere in which elders may feel encouraged and respected. Foster an inclusive and accepting atmosphere in which everyone, regardless of age or ability, is welcome. Create chances for peer support and mentorship to instill a sense of belonging and accountability.

Overall, building a supportive exercise environment for elders to lose weight involves meticulous preparation, attention to detail, and a dedication to promoting a positive and inclusive environment. By addressing physical, social, and psychological components, you may help elders adopt an active lifestyle and reach their fitness objectives.

I am committed to putting my fitness and health everyday first

CHAPTER TWO

Flexibility Training for Seniors

Flexibility exercises serve to maintain joint mobility, lower the chance of injury, and enhance the general quality of life. For seniors aiming to reduce weight, adding flexibility exercise into their regimen is critical to meeting their fitness objectives.

Begin your flexibility training with simple warm-up activities that will boost blood flow to your muscles and prepare your body for stretching. Simple exercises like arm circles, shoulder rolls, and moderate neck stretches are excellent choices.

Stretch key muscular groups including your calves, hamstrings, quadriceps, hips, back, chest, shoulders, and arms. Hold each stretch for 15 to 30 seconds, inhaling deeply and relaxing into it. Remember not to bounce or push the stretch, and never extend so far that you feel discomfort.

Include a range of flexibility exercises in your program, such as yoga, Pilates, and tai chi, to keep things fresh and target different muscle areas. These exercises also assist seniors improve their balance and coordination, which are crucial skills.

Make flexibility training a regular element of your fitness program, with at least 2-3 sessions each week. Consistency is essential for gradually improving your flexibility.

Pay attention to your body and adjust routines to meet any physical restrictions or health issues. If you're not sure whether workouts are safe for you, speak with a fitness expert or physical therapist.

Flexibility training is an important aspect of fitness for seniors, particularly those who want to reduce weight. Regular stretching exercises can increase joint mobility, lower the chance of injury, and improve your general health. Remember to start cautiously, listen to your body, and maintain consistency in your practice.

Benefits of Flexibility Exercises

Flexibility exercises are essential for seniors who want to shed weight and maintain good health. For starters, they improve joint range of motion, which reduces the likelihood of damage during athletic activity. Stretching frequently helps your muscles become more elastic, allowing you to move more easily and comfortably.

Second, flexibility exercises enhance posture and balance. As we age, our posture deteriorates, resulting in imbalances and probable falls. Exercises like yoga and Pilates assist in rectifying posture by strengthening core muscles and encouraging alignment. Better balance leads to fewer accidents and greater confidence in daily tasks.

Furthermore, flexibility exercises reduce muscular tension and pain. Stretching promotes blood flow to the muscles, which aids in the clearance of toxins and reduces stiffness. This promotes faster recovery after exercise and reduces the probability of muscular cramping or soreness.

Including flexibility exercises in your program improves general mobility and functionality. Improved flexibility allows you to complete daily chores more effectively, such as bending, reaching, and lifting. This freedom is essential for sustaining a good standard of living as you age.

Flexibility exercises have also been linked to improved mental wellness. They induce relaxation and alleviate stress by releasing tension from the body. This can result in improved sleep quality and general well-being, both of which are necessary for optimal weight management.

Flexibility exercises have several benefits for seniors wanting to lose weight. They contribute significantly to developing and sustaining a healthy lifestyle by improving joint mobility, posture, and balance, relieving muscular stress, boosting general mobility, and fostering mental well-being.

Incorporating these exercises into your fitness program can result in considerable benefits in both physical and mental health.

Upper Body Stretching Techniques

To successfully stretch your upper body, begin with easy movements that target specific muscle groups. Begin by standing tall, shoulder-width apart.

Neck Stretch: Gently tilt your head to one side, moving your ear closer to your shoulder, until you feel a stretch on the opposite side of your neck. Hold for 15-30 seconds then swap sides.

Shoulder Stretch: Bring one arm across your body and use the opposing hand to gently push the elbow into your chest until you feel a stretch in your shoulder. Hold for 15-30 seconds then swap sides.

Triceps Stretch: Extend one arm above, bending at the elbow and reaching down the middle of the back. With the opposite hand, gently press on the elbow, feeling the stretch around the back of your arm. Hold for 15-30 seconds then swap sides.

Chest Stretch: Interlace your fingers behind your back, straighten your arms, and elevate them slightly away from your body. Feel the strain on your chest and shoulders. Hold for 15–30 seconds.

Upper back stretch: Place your hands together in front of you, palms facing outward. Round your upper back, moving your hands away from your body and lowering your chin to your chest. Hold for 15–30 seconds.

Arm Circles: Extend your arms out to the sides, shoulder height. Make tiny circles with your arms, gradually increasing the size of each circle. After 10-15 seconds, reverse direction.

These stretches may be adjusted to suit seniors' fitness levels and mobility. Encourage them to do these stretches every day to increase flexibility, reduce stiffness, and encourage improved posture.

To avoid injury, always highlight the significance of appropriate breathing and body awareness. As they get more comfortable, they can progressively extend the time of each stretch to maximize their benefits.

Lower Body Stretching Techniques

When it comes to lower-body stretching exercises, flexibility and mobility should be prioritized, especially for seniors who want to lose weight. To warm up your muscles and boost blood flow. Start with active stretches like hip circles and leg swings

After that, do static stretches for key muscular groups such as the quadriceps, hamstrings, calves, and glutes. A standing quad stretch involves raising one foot towards your buttocks while keeping balance and holding onto a sturdy surface as needed.

Hold the stretch for 15-30 seconds, then swap sides.

To stretch your hamstrings, sit on the ground with one leg extended and the other bowed. Reach for your toes while maintaining your back straight and feel the stretch at the back of your leg. Hold for 15-30 seconds then swap legs.

For the calves, face a wall with one-foot front and the other back, both heels on the ground. Until you feel a stretch in the calf of your rear leg, continue learning forward

Hold for 15-30 seconds then swap legs. For the glutes, sit on the ground with one leg bent and the other crossed over, hugging the bent knee close to your chest.

Breathe deeply and relax into each stretch, avoiding any bouncing motions that may result in harm. Aim to include these stretches into your routine at least 2-3 times each week, progressively increasing the duration and intensity as your flexibility grows. Stretching your lower body daily not only improves mobility and reduces the chance of injury, but it also helps you lose weight by increasing total muscle function and efficiency during exercise.

Core Flexibility Exercises

To improve core flexibility, focus on workouts that target the muscles that surround your abdominal, lower back, and pelvis. Engaging in a balanced routine will enhance mobility, stability, and posture, which are essential for everyday tasks and reduce the chance of injury.

Warm up your muscles by doing mild stretches like pelvic tilts and trunk rotations. These motions relieve tension and prepare the body for deeper stretches. As your flexibility improves, gradually increase the difficulty of your workouts.

Incorporate dynamic motions, such as leg swings and arm circles, to improve fluidity and enhance range of motion. These exercises increase blood flow to the muscles, which aids in healing and flexibility.

To extend and relieve tension in the muscles surrounding your spine, use static stretches such as the cat-cow stretch and the sitting spinal twist. Hold each stretch for 15-30 seconds, then breathe deeply to deepen the stretch and relax your muscles.

Use equipment such as stability balls and resistance bands to provide variation and intensity to your workout. Stability ball exercises like the plank and bridge work many muscle groups at once, increasing core strength and flexibility.

Resistance bands offer support across the whole range of action, therefore increasing muscular flexibility and strength.

To improve efficacy and avoid injury, maintain perfect form and alignment during each exercise. Listen to your body and adjust routines to meet any physical restrictions or pain.

Consistency is essential for seeing benefits, so strive to do core flexibility exercises at least 2-3 times each week. Combine these workouts with cardiovascular activity and a well-balanced diet to help you lose weight and improve your health.

Before beginning any new fitness regimen, speak with a healthcare practitioner, especially if you have pre-existing health ailments or concerns. Stay hydrated, listen to your body, and enjoy the path to greater core flexibility and general well-being.

Integrated Flexibility Routine

Integrated flexibility workouts aim to improve general flexibility while including movements that stimulate numerous muscle groups at once. For seniors looking to reduce weight, these workouts provide a mild yet efficient way to improve mobility while burning calories.

Begin with a modest warm-up, such as walking or light cardio, to prepare your body for activity. For main muscle groups such as torso twists, arm circles and leg swings, dynamic Stretches should be integrated

These activities improve blood flow and flexibility while lowering the chance of injury.

Transition to integrated activities that incorporate flexibility and strength training. Examples include lunges with a twist, which include lunging forward while rotating your torso to activate the core and stretch the hips.

Another alternative is the bird-dog exercise, which includes extending one arm and the opposing leg while balancing on all fours to improve overall body stability and flexibility.

To get the most out of the practice and encourage relaxation, focus on smooth movements and regulated breathing. As you develop, progressively increase the intensity and length of each workout while listening to your body and staying within your boundaries.

Incorporate stretches for particular areas of stiffness or discomfort, such as the hamstrings, hips, and shoulders. Hold each stretch for 15-30 seconds, concentrating on deep breathing and relaxation to relieve tension and increase flexibility.

Finish the workout with a cooldown that includes static stretches to improve flexibility and recovery. Calf stretches, quad stretches, and shoulder stretches, all of which are held for 30-60 seconds to enable the muscles to relax and extend.

Focus is essential for seeing benefits, so include this integrated flexibility practice into your weekly calendar, gradually increasing the frequency and intensity as you feel comfortable.

Consult a healthcare expert before beginning any new fitness regimen, especially if you have pre-existing health ailments or concerns.

With perseverance and patience, you may reap the advantages of increased flexibility and weight loss far into your retirement years.

With every workout I am putting my long time progress first

CHAPTER THREE

Core Strength Exercises for Seniors

As a senior, focus on modest yet effective core strengthening activities. Start with sitting core exercises like knee raises and torso twists. These exercises work the core muscles while avoiding tension on the back or hips.

Next, integrate standing core workouts such as knee lifts and side bends. These activities promote balance and stability while strengthening the core muscles.

Another useful exercise is the plank, which may be adapted for seniors by doing it on an elevated platform like a chair or countertop. Hold the plank position for as long as you feel comfortable, progressively increasing the duration over time.

Do not underestimate the value of flexibility exercises for elders. Stretching the core muscles, such as seated forward bends and seated spinal twists, can assist increase range of motion and lower the risk of injury.

Oblique twists and side plank variants are also important exercises to incorporate. These exercises serve to strengthen the muscles that twist and rotate the torso.

Walking, swimming, and tai chi, in addition to particular core workouts, can help seniors improve their general core strength and fitness levels. These low-impact workouts deliver a full-body workout while being easy on your joints.

Importance of Core Strength for Seniors

As you become older, having strong core muscles becomes increasingly important for your general health and functionality. Your core muscles, which include your abdominal, lower back, pelvis, and hips, give stability and support during everyday activities like walking, bending, and lifting.

Strengthening these muscles can help to improve balance and minimize the chance of falling, which is especially essential for seniors. A strong core can also reduce back discomfort and improve posture, increasing your quality of life and independence.

Seniors should include core-strengthening activities in their fitness program. Planks, bridges, and sitting twists are good exercises for targeting the core muscles without placing too much effort on other portions of the body.

These exercises may be tailored to your fitness level and skills, making them accessible and safe for seniors with varying degrees of mobility.

Working on core strength might help seniors lose and control their weight. A strong core promotes appropriate alignment during exercise, resulting in increased calorie burn and efficient movement patterns.

A strong core can increase overall metabolic performance, resulting in more efficient fat-burning and weight reduction over time.

When starting a core-strengthening regimen, it's critical to begin softly and progressively increase intensity and length as your strength grows. Consistency is important, so integrate core workouts into your program at least twice to three times each week for the best results.

Always ensure to pay attention to your body and speak with a fitness expert if you have any concerns or limits.

By including core strength into your training routine, you will not only improve your physical health and functionality as a senior but also your general well-being and quality of life.

So, take the time to strengthen your core muscles today for a healthier, happier tomorrow.

Core Activation Techniques

Seniors might benefit from a variety of strategies suited to their specific needs for optimum core activation. Begin by stimulating your deep abdominal muscles, such as the transverse abdominis, with diaphragmatic breathing exercises.

Inhale deeply, extending your abdomen, and then exhale fully, pushing your belly button closer to your spine. This not only works your core, but it also improves good posture and stability.

Next, integrate exercises that work for many muscular groups at once, such as planks or bird dogs. These exercises test your core stability while simultaneously working your arms, legs, and back muscles. Begin with modified versions if necessary, such as planks on your knees or bird dogs with a chair for support.

Use stability balls or resistance bands to increase the variety and intensity of your workouts. To strengthen your core while sitting or standing, try seated stability ball marches or resistance band woodchops.

These gadgets offer modest resistance, making them suitable for seniors who want to gain strength without risking harm. Prioritize balance and coordination workouts to strengthen your core muscles.

Simple tasks like standing on one leg or walking heel to toe not only strengthen your core but also enhance your general stability and lower your chance of falling.

Do not underestimate the value of excellent form and technique. During your workouts, keep your spine neutral and prevent excessive arching or rounding of the back.

Use your core muscles carefully with each action, and remember to breathe steadily to support your efforts. Core activation for seniors consists of deep abdominal engagement, multi-muscle movements, stability and resistance training, balancing drills, and mindful technique.

By combining these exercises into your training program, you may successfully strengthen your core, increase general stability, and help with weight reduction in a safe and controlled way.

Abdominal Strengthening Exercises

Exercise diversity improves general health and well-being in addition to strengthening your core.

Crunches: Start by bending your knees while resting on your back. Elevate your upper body while maintaining a relaxed neck and a slightly tucked chin. With control, lower yourself back down. Aim for two to three sets of ten to fifteen repetitions.

Leg Raises: Maintaining your legs straight, raise both of your legs toward the ceiling while lying flat on your back. Gently return them to the ground without making contact with it. Repeat for two to three sets of ten to twelve repetitions.

Planks: Take a push-up stance, but instead of using your hands to support your weight, use your forearms. Engage your core muscles and maintain a straight body alignment from head to heels. Hold for 20 to 30 seconds at a time, extending the time as you go.

Russian Twists: Bend your knees while sitting on the floor with your feet raised off the floor. Slightly recline your head and turn your torso such that each side touches the ground. On each side, try to get two to three sets of 12 to 15 twists.

Hands on the sides of the chair to provide support when you sit down for seated knee tucks. Using your core muscles, bring your knees up to your chest. Carefully lower them back down.

Do 2–3 sets of 10–12 repetitions.

Throughout every exercise, pay close attention to your breathing and technique to increase efficiency and reduce the chance of injury. Furthermore, pay attention to your body and move at a comfortable yet demanding speed.

For best effects, try to include these workouts in your regimen at least twice or three times a week. Consistency is the key.

Be sure to drink enough water, eat a well-balanced diet, and see a doctor before beginning any new fitness program, particularly if you have any underlying medical issues.

You'll be well on your way to reaching your fitness objectives and leading a more active, healthy lifestyle with commitment and perseverance.

Back Strengthening Exercises

Simple yet effective workouts are essential for strengthening your back and promoting weight reduction. Begin with bodyweight exercises like bird dogs, which work the lower back muscles and enhance stability. Next, attempt bridges to work your glutes and lower back while training your core muscles.

Moving on, incorporate Superman exercises into your regimen to strengthen your entire back, including the muscles along your spine. This exercise improves posture and lowers the chance of back problems. Sitting rows with resistance bands or cable machines efficiently target upper back muscles, improving total back strength and stability.

Modified workouts for seniors, such as sitting rows with resistance bands or machine help, can be more easy on the joints while still offering a useful workout. Adding these exercises to your program two to three times per week might result in visible improvements in back strength and posture over time.

Don't underestimate the value of stretching exercises for improving flexibility and preventing stiffness in your back. Include stretches like cat-cow and child's pose in your regimen to relieve tension and encourage relaxation in your back muscles.

Give attention to your body and begin with less resistance or fewer repetitions if necessary. Gradually up the intensity and volume as your strength and endurance improve. Before beginning any new workout program, contact with a fitness expert or healthcare practitioner, especially if you have a history of back problems or accidents.

By including these back-strengthening exercises into your routine and sticking to a consistent training regimen, you may help with weight reduction while also improving general back health and function.

Total Core Strength Workout Routine

To improve your overall core strength, use a well-rounded workout plan that targets all muscle groups in your core area. Begin with basic exercises like planks, which work your whole core, including your abdominals, obliques, and lower back muscles. Hold the plank posture for 30-60 seconds, progressively increasing the time as your strength improves.

Include exercises that target multiple angles of your core, such as Russian twists for the obliques and bicycle crunches for the rectus abdominis. For each exercise, aim for 2-3 sets of 12-15 repetitions while maintaining perfect technique.

Use stability ball workouts to increase the challenge and improve balance. Try stability ball rollouts to work your deep core muscles and stability ball crunches to activate your abdominals while keeping your body stable on the ball.

Don't overlook your lower back muscles, since they play an important part in total core strength and stability. Use exercises like Superman holds, bridges, and deadlifts to strengthen your lower back and prevent imbalances.

Incorporate functional motions that are similar to regular tasks to increase total core strength and functioning. Standing wood chops, bird dogs, and standing cable rotations are all exercises that work for many muscular groups while requiring core stability.

Seniors who want to reduce weight should focus on workouts that are easy on their joints while yet burning calories. Incorporate low-impact cardio workouts such as walking, swimming, or cycling into your daily routine to improve cardiovascular health and burn calories.

Combine aerobic workouts with strength training routines that target all major muscle groups, including the core, to increase lean muscle mass and metabolism. Aim for at least 150 minutes of moderate-intensity cardio and 2-3 days of strength training each week for the best benefits.

I wholeheartedly accept the benefits and Movements it brings to my life

CHAPTER FOUR

Balance and Stability Training

Balance and stability training is crucial for seniors looking to lose weight and maintain overall health. As you age, your balance naturally declines, increasing the risk of falls and injuries.

By incorporating balance and stability exercises into your routine, you not only improve your physical abilities but also enhance your confidence and independence.

Start with simple exercises that focus on strengthening your core muscles, such as standing on one leg or performing seated leg lifts. These exercises help improve proprioception, which is your body's awareness of its position in space.

Incorporate balance tools like stability balls, balance boards, or foam pads to challenge your stability further. These tools force your body to engage stabilizing muscles, improving your balance over time.

Tai chi and yoga are excellent options for seniors, as they combine balance, strength, and flexibility exercises in one practice. These low-impact activities not only improve physical stability but also promote mental well-being and relaxation.

Include dynamic movements that mimic everyday activities, such as walking heel-to-toe or stepping over obstacles. These functional exercises help you maintain balance in real-life situations, reducing the risk of falls.

Consistency is key. Aim for at least 2-3 balance and stability sessions per week, gradually increasing intensity and difficulty as you progress.

Include balance training into your existing fitness routine or dedicate specific days to focus solely on balance and stability. Mix it up to keep things interesting and challenge different muscle groups.

Always prioritize safety. Perform exercises near a sturdy surface or have a chair nearby for support if needed. Stay hydrated and wear supportive footwear to prevent slips and falls.

Through balance and stability training into your fitness routine, you not only improve your physical health but also enhance your quality of life as you age. Stay committed, stay consistent, and enjoy the benefits of a stronger, more stable body.

Importance of Balance Training for Seniors

Balance training is important for seniors because it helps avoid falls, which can result in catastrophic injuries. As you become older, your balance gradually deteriorates owing to muscular weakening and changes in eyesight and proprioception. By including balancing exercises in your regimen, you may enhance stability and lower your chance of falling.

One significant advantage of balancing training is its improved effect on total functional abilities. As you improve the muscles involved in balance, you will be able to do daily actions like walking, climbing stairs, and reaching for things more steadily.

Additionally, balance training improves proprioception, or your body's sense of its location in space. This increased awareness allows you to respond more rapidly to changes in your surroundings, minimizing the danger of falling.

Balancing exercises promote muscular activation across the body, resulting in enhanced muscle tone and strength. This can also help with weight reduction and general fitness since it increases calorie expenditure and promotes lean muscle mass growth.

Incorporating balance exercises into seniors' workout routines might help them lose weight. While balance training alone may not result in considerable weight loss, it is an important part of supporting overall health and fitness objectives.

Standing on one leg, walking heel-to-toe, and doing tai chi or yoga positions that emphasize stability and coordination are all simple balancing exercises appropriate for seniors. These exercises are readily adapted to meet individual fitness levels and may be done at home or in a group environment.

Balance training is vital for seniors who want to retain stability, avoid falls, and enhance their general functional capacity. Incorporating balance exercises into your daily routine, along with other types of physical activity, can help you lose weight while also improving your health and well-being.

Static Balance Exercises

Static balancing exercises are an excellent choice for seniors looking to lose weight through simple workout activities. These exercises improve stability while simultaneously engaging core muscles, encouraging calorie burn and weight reduction.

To begin, integrate basic static balancing exercises into your program. Begin with the fundamental stance: stand tall, feet hip-width apart, and distribute your weight evenly. Maintain equilibrium by using your core muscles and focusing on a fixed point ahead.

Make progress by testing your equilibrium further. Try standing on one leg and keeping an appropriate posture. Lift one foot off the ground slightly to keep your standing leg steady. Hold this posture for as long as you feel comfortable, to gradually increase the duration.

The tandem stance is yet another great static balancing exercise. Position one foot exactly in front of the other, heel to toe, keeping your balance without wavering. Focus on a point in front of you to help with stability, and hold for as long as possible.

To enhance the diversity and complexity of your exercise, use balance-enhancing props such as stability balls or balance boards. These instruments create an unstable surface, making your muscles work harder to maintain stability.

Static balancing exercises require a high level of consistency. Aim for at least 10-15 minutes of practice many times each week to observe significant gains in balance and weight loss. As you grow, push yourself with longer holds or more challenging versions to keep reaping the advantages.

Dynamic Balance Exercises

Dynamic balancing exercises are essential for seniors trying to shed weight and improve their general health. These exercises improve stability and coordination by exercising numerous muscle groups.

Begin with easy exercises such as leg swings, which include standing and swinging one leg forward and backward, then side to side. This activity tests your balance and activates your leg muscles.

Lift one foot off the ground and hold it there for 10-30 seconds before moving on to single-leg standing. This exercise increases ankle stability and general balance.

Incorporate weight-shifting motions like side lunges and lateral leg lifts. These exercises push your body to steady while moving, which improves dynamic balance.

Use balancing boards or stability balls to offer an added challenge. workouts such as sitting ball passes or standing on a balancing board while performing arm workouts. These instruments cause your body to stabilize, which improves balance and coordination.

Include tasks that simulate real-life motions, such as walking heel-to-toe or stepping over obstacles. These useful workouts help people improve their balance in regular tasks.

Participate in tai chi or yoga, which emphasize slow, controlled motions that require balance and flexibility. These techniques not only improve physical balance but also increase mental clarity and calm.

Consistency is essential; strive to include dynamic balancing exercises in your regimen at least 2-3 times each week. Start with 10-15 minutes and progressively increase the time and intensity as you go.

Always put safety first by having robust support nearby and wearing suitable footwear. Listen to your body and alter routines as necessary to avoid damage.

Seniors who do dynamic balancing exercises daily can enhance their stability, coordination, and general fitness while working toward weight loss objectives.

Proprioception Training

Proprioception training is essential for seniors wanting to reduce weight with simple fitness workouts. Proprioception is your body's capacity to detect its location in space and the relative positions of its components without using eyesight.

This exercise improves balance, coordination, and total body awareness, lowering the likelihood of falls and injuries associated with aging.

To begin, use easy balancing exercises in your program. Begin by standing on one leg for longer durations, progressively testing yourself. Use balancing boards or foam cushions to increase difficulty. These exercises activate your proprioceptive system, which increases stability and core strength.

Next, incorporate functional motions that simulate everyday tasks. Squats, lunges, and step-ups enhance balance and strength while working several muscle groups. Performing these motions with good form improves proprioception by requiring your body to adapt and stabilize.

To test your proprioceptive talents even further, use agility workouts. Side shuffles, grapevines, and ladder drills can help you enhance your dynamic balance and coordination.

These workouts mimic real-life motions, improving your body's capacity to react and adapt to changing circumstances.

Also, integrate unstable surfaces into your routines. Use stability balls, Bosu balls, or balance discs for workouts like push-ups, planks, and leg lifts. These technologies create an unstable environment, requiring your body to use stabilizing muscles and increase proprioception.

Consider hobbies like tai chi or yoga, which stress calm, controlled movements, and conscious body awareness. These routines improve proprioception while also encouraging relaxation and stress reduction.

Consistency is essential in proprioception training. Aim to do at least 2-3 sessions each week, progressively increasing the intensity and complexity as you advance. Remember to listen to your body and move at your speed to avoid injury.

By including proprioception training into your workout routine, you will not only improve balance and coordination but also increase total body awareness, which will help you lose weight as a senior.

Complete Balance Workout Plan

To construct a well-rounded workout schedule, include activities that target many aspects of fitness, such as cardiovascular endurance, strength, flexibility, and balance. Start with a 5-10 minute warm-up to get your body ready for a workout. This might be quick walking, marching in place, or light stretching.

To improve cardiovascular endurance, strive for at least 30 minutes of moderate-intensity aerobic activity most days of the week. This might include walking, swimming, riding, or dancing. As your fitness level increases, gradually increase the time and intensity.

Strength exercise is essential for seniors to keep their muscle mass and bone density. Include activities that target all main muscular groups, such as squats, lunges, push-ups, and rowing. Use resistance bands or modest weights to safely work your muscles. Aim for 2-3 sessions each week, with a day of recovery in between.

Flexibility exercises assist in preserving the range of motion and avoiding injury. Incorporate mild stretches for all main muscle groups, holding them for 15-30 seconds without bouncing. Yoga or tai chi sessions can also help you improve your flexibility and balance.

Speaking of balance, it's critical to incorporate activities that test your stability and coordination. Consider standing on one leg, walking heel-to-toe, or doing yoga positions such as tree pose or warrior III. Aim for 2-3 sessions each week to improve balance and lower your chance of falling.

Don't stop listening to your body and adjust the workouts as required. Stay hydrated, and don't forget to cool down with some mild stretching after your workout. Consistency is crucial, so make exercise a regular part of your schedule.

My body is capable, resilient and strong In bringing Positive change to my life

CHAPTER FIVE

Sample Workouts for Seniors

Seniors wishing to reduce weight with simple fitness routines should select low-impact activities that nevertheless give a solid workout. Here's a complete guide to example workouts designed exclusively for seniors:

Walking: Begin with at least 30 minutes of brisk walking five days a week. As your fitness level increases, gradually increase the time and intensity.

Swimming: Swimming is easy on the joints and provides a full-body workout. Aim for 20-30 minutes of swimming laps with appropriate form and rhythm iding: Whether on a stationary bike or outside, riding is beneficial to cardiovascular health and leg strength. Begin with 15-20 minutes and progressively increase duration and resistance.

Chair Exercises: To develop strength and flexibility while sitting, use sat exercises such as leg lifts, arm curls with low weights, and seated marches.

Yoga encourages balance, flexibility, and relaxation. Look for beginner-friendly workshops or DVDs that emphasize gentle stretches and postures appropriate for elders. Tai Chi combines soft motions with deep breathing to improve balance, coordination, and overall well-being.

Join a class or watch online videos to master the fundamentals.

Resistance training involves using resistance bands or small weights to conduct workouts that target main muscle groups. Begin with 1-2 sets of 10-12 repetitions per exercise, gradually increasing the intensity over time.

Simple balance exercises, such as standing on one leg, heel-to-toe walks, or Stay hydrated, warm and avoid falling.up before exercising, and cool down afterward to avoid injury. Consistency is crucial, so incorporate exercise into your daily routine for long-term weight loss and general health advantages.

Beginner's Workout Routine

Begin with a simple warm-up to prepare your muscles and joints. Consider 5-10 minutes of brisk walking or modest cardio activity, such as stationary cycling. This prepares your body for the forthcoming activity and lowers the danger of damage.

Next, concentrate on strength-training exercises. Begin with bodyweight exercises like squats, lunges, wall pushups, and seated leg lifts.

For 10-15 repetitions per exercise, aim for 2-3 sets

These activities assist develop muscular mass and increase metabolism, which aids in weight reduction.

Use resistance bands or light dumbbells to progressively increase the intensity as you develop. Remember to use good form to avoid strain.

After strength training, do some balance and flexibility exercises. Tai chi, yoga, or basic balance drills like standing on one leg help enhance stability and reduce falls, which are significant concerns among seniors.

Set aside time for aerobic activity to increase your heart rate and burn calories. Choose low-impact activities such as swimming, water aerobics, or brisk strolling. Aim for at least 20-30 minutes of cardio every day, increasing the time and intensity as your fitness increases.

Cool down with stretches that target main muscle groups. Hold each stretch for 15-30 seconds, concentrating on deep breathing and relaxing into the stretch. This helps to minimize muscular pain and increase flexibility.

Aim for at least three to four workouts each week, increasing the frequency and intensity as you feel comfortable.
Before beginning any new workout program, consult with a fitness expert or your healthcare practitioner, especially if you have any underlying health issues.

Intermediate Exercise Plan

Begin with an active warm-up to get your muscles and joints ready for exercise. Include workouts that progressively raise your heart rate, such as brisk walking, cycling, or swimming, for at least 30 minutes five days a week.

Incorporate resistance training routines with light dumbbells or resistance bands to increase muscular growth and metabolism. Squats, lunges, push-ups, and rows are excellent full-body exercises for targeting key muscle groups and developing functional strength and balance.

Aim for two to three sessions each week, with appropriate recuperation between workouts.

Include flexibility exercises, such as yoga or stretching regimens, to improve mobility and avoid injury. Perform static stretches for each major muscle group, holding them for 15-30 seconds without bouncing, preferably after your workout or during cooldown.

Include balance exercises in your regimen to lessen the danger of falling and improve stability. To test your balance and coordination, try standing on one leg, heel-to-toe walks, or Tai Chi exercises.

Aim for two to three sessions each week, progressively increasing the length and difficulty of the exercises as you advance.

Listen to your body and modify the intensity and length of your workouts based on your fitness level and any underlying medical concerns. To achieve the best outcomes, stay hydrated, eat nutrient-dense meals, and prioritize appropriate rest and recuperation time.

Advanced Fitness Program

Begin with a vigorous warm-up exercise to get your body ready for more strenuous workouts. Include movements such as arm circles, leg swings, and slow running in place for 5-10 minutes. This improves blood flow to your muscles and lowers the danger of damage.

Next, concentrate on strength training routines that use resistance bands or small weights. Exercises for key muscular areas include squats, lunges, chest presses, rows, and shoulder presses.

Progressively increasing the weight as you go, aim for 2-3 sets of 10-15 repetitions on every exercise

Incorporate cardiovascular exercises to increase your heart rate and burn calories efficiently. Brisk walking, cycling, swimming, and the use of cardio devices such as ellipticals or stationary cycles are all options. Aim for at least 30 minutes of moderate-intensity exercise on most days of the week.

Don't forget about flexibility and balance exercises, which are essential for keeping mobility and avoiding falls. Include stretches for all main muscle groups, holding each for 15 to 30 seconds. Practice balance exercises such as standing on one leg or utilizing stability balls to test your stability.

Integrate high-intensity interval training (HIIT) to increase calorie burn and overall fitness. Alternate short bursts of intensive activity (such as running or jumping jacks) with brief intervals of relaxation. Begin with 20-30 seconds of effort, followed by 10-20 seconds of rest. Repeat for 5-10 rounds.

Prioritize recovery and rest days to enable your body to heal and strengthen. To support your fitness objectives, make sure you get enough sleep, remain hydrated, and eat nutritional meals.

Chair-Based Workout Options

To begin, consider integrating sitting cardio workouts such as sat marching or seated leg lifts to increase your heart rate and burn calories effectively. These exercises may be done in a chair, which provides stability and reduces joint stress.

Next, focus on strength training with resistance bands or light dumbbells for sitting arm curls, shoulder presses, and leg extensions. Strengthening your muscles not only helps you lose weight, but it also improves your balance and lowers your chance of injury.

Incorporate chair yoga or stretching practices to increase flexibility, circulation, and relieve tension. These low-impact workouts are mild on the body yet extremely useful to overall health.

Do not forget about core workouts! Seated abdominal twists and pelvic tilts can help tone your core and improve posture, resulting in a slimmer profile.

To keep things interesting, try taking chair-based fitness courses tailored exclusively for elders. These sessions frequently involve a range of motions to target certain muscle regions while also offering social connection and motivation.

Always listen to your body and alter activities based on your fitness level and any pre-existing issues. Consistency is essential, so integrate chair-based workouts into your regimen many times each week for best results.

To help you lose weight, stay hydrated, eat a balanced diet rich in whole foods, and make sure you get enough rest and recuperation time. With effort and determination, you may reach your fitness objectives and enjoy better health and energy throughout your golden years.

Quick and Efficient Exercise Routines

For seniors looking to lose weight, short and effective workout programs are essential. Use a combination of aerobic and strength training activities to increase calorie burn and muscle mass, which boosts metabolism.

Begin with a 5- to 10-minute warm-up to prepare your body and avoid injuries. Walking, mild cycling, and arm circles are all possible options.

Incorporate interval training into your program. To optimize calorie expenditure, alternate between high-intensity bursts and low-intensity or rest intervals. Examples include walking and running alternately, as well as riding at different speeds.

Incorporate strength training workouts to develop muscle and boost metabolism. Concentrate on complex exercises such as squats, lunges, push-ups, and rows. For 8-12 repetitions per exercise, aim to get 2-3 sets.

For ease and safety, use bodyweight exercises like squats, lunges, push-ups, and planks. Integrate balance and flexibility activities such as yoga, tai chi, or basic balance exercises to increase stability and mobility.

Finish with 5-10 minutes of stretching to improve flexibility and relieve muscular pain. Stretch all main muscle groups, holding each for 15-30 seconds.

Consistency is essential for success. Aim for at least 30 minutes of moderate-intensity activity most days of the week, including at least two days of strength training. Listen to your body and modify activities as needed to avoid damage.

Stay hydrated and nourish your body with nutritional foods to help you achieve your fitness and weight reduction objectives.

Before beginning any new workout plan, contact a fitness expert or your healthcare practitioner, especially if you have any underlying health issues.

Every move I make brings me closer to the health i desire

CHAPTER SIX

Nutrition Tips for Seniors

Prioritize Nutrient-Dense Foods: Include nutrient-dense foods like fruits, vegetables, lean meats, whole grains, and healthy fats in your diet. These foods include the vital vitamins, minerals, and antioxidants required for good health.

Stay Hydrated: As you age, your feeling of thirst may diminish, resulting in dehydration. Drink enough water throughout the day to keep your body hydrated and functioning properly.

Portion Control: Pay attention to portion proportions to avoid overeating, which can lead to weight gain. Smaller plates and bowls might help you regulate your quantities and avoid eating too many calories.

Limit Processed Meals and Added Sugars: Reduce your intake of processed meals, sugary snacks, and beverages, since they provide little nutritious value and can contribute to weight gain and other health problems.

Include Calcium and Vitamin D in Your Diet: To promote bone health, incorporate calcium-rich foods such as dairy products, leafy greens, and fortified meals. For maximum absorption, combine these meals with vitamin D sources such as fatty fish and sunshine.

Reduce Your Sodium Intake: Limit your intake of processed and packaged foods, use fresh ingredients, and season meals with herbs and spices rather than salt.

Listen to Your Body: Be aware of hunger and fullness cues, and eat thoughtfully. Avoid distractions when eating and take your time enjoying each bite. Now, let's talk about some basic fitness routines for seniors to help them lose weight:

Walking: Begin with short walks and progressively increase the time and intensity. Walking is low-impact, gentle on the joints, and can be done in almost any place.

Water Aerobics: Take a water aerobics class or do water workouts in the pool. Water offers resistance while supporting the body, making it an excellent choice for elders.

Chair Yoga: Practice mild yoga postures and stretches while sitting in a chair. Chair yoga increases flexibility, strength, and balance without placing strain on joints.

Resistance Band Workouts: Use resistance band exercises to gain muscle and boost metabolism. These exercises may be tailored to any fitness level and are mild on the joints.

Combining these eating guidelines with frequent physical activity can help you control your weight and enhance your overall health and well-being as a senior.

Importance of Nutrition for Older Adults

As you age, your body's nutritional demands vary, necessitating an emphasis on nutrient-dense meals to promote general health and well-being. Adequate nutrition is required to maintain muscular mass, bone density, cognitive function, and immunological function, all of which play important roles in good aging.

Older persons must prioritize nutrient-dense foods including fruits, vegetables, lean meats, whole grains, and healthy fats. These foods provide vital vitamins, minerals, antioxidants, and fiber, which support a variety of biological processes and protect against chronic illnesses linked with aging, such as heart disease, diabetes, and osteoporosis.

An appropriate diet can help with weight management by regulating hunger, increasing satiety, and maintaining metabolic health. Seniors who want to reduce weight should focus on developing a balanced eating plan that includes a range of meals from all food categories while regulating portion sizes and limiting consumption of processed and high-calorie items.

In addition to eating, integrating simple fitness workouts into your regimen can aid in weight reduction and general wellness. Walking, swimming, cycling, and tai chi are low-impact exercises that are easy on the joints while offering significant cardiovascular and strength-building benefits.

Strength training with small weights or resistance bands can assist enhance muscle mass and bone density, both of which decrease with age. These exercises may be tailored to specific fitness levels and skills, making them suitable for older individuals of different ages and physical ailments.

Maintaining a healthy lifestyle in your senior years is about more than just looking and feeling well; it's also about retaining independence and enjoying a great quality of life.

 Prioritizing diet and implementing simple fitness workouts into your regimen will help you age well and stay healthy.

Balanced Meal Planning for Weight Loss

When preparing balanced meals for weight reduction, prioritize nutrient-dense foods that will meet your body's needs while producing a calorie deficit.

Begin by using lean proteins such as chicken, fish, tofu, or beans in your meals to encourage satiety and muscle restoration.

Protein should be combined with high-fiber carbs like whole grains, fruits, and vegetables to help regulate blood sugar levels and keep you feeling fuller for longer.

To promote cell function and satiety, choose healthy fats such as olive oil, almonds and avocado.

Divide your meal into three sections: half with non-starchy veggies like leafy greens, peppers, and broccoli; one quarter with lean protein; and one quarter with healthy grains or starchy vegetables like sweet potatoes or quinoa.

This balanced approach guarantees that you receive a range of nutrients while keeping portion amounts under control. To supplement your eating plan, include simple fitness workouts for seniors to help in weight loss.

Low-impact sports such as walking, swimming, and cycling can help you improve your cardiovascular health and burn calories without placing too much strain on your joints. Strength training with small weights or resistance bands can help maintain muscle mass and enhance metabolism, resulting in long-term weight reduction success.

Incorporate flexibility and balance activities, such as yoga or tai chi, to increase mobility and minimize the chance of falls, which are prevalent among seniors.

Aim for at least 150 minutes of moderate-intensity aerobic activity or 75 minutes of intense activity each week, with two days of strength and balance exercises.

Nutrient-Rich Foods for Seniors

As you age, your body's nutritional requirements vary, necessitating a concentration of nutrient-dense foods to maintain general health and vigor.
which

First and foremost, make fruits and vegetables a priority in your diet. These foods are high in important vitamins, minerals, and antioxidants, which help prevent age-related disorders and increase longevity. Aim to fill half of your plate with bright fruits and veggies at every meal.

Next, incorporate lean protein sources including fish, chicken, eggs, beans, and lentils. Protein is essential for preserving muscle mass, tends to decrease with age.

Protein-rich meals also help you feel full and satisfied, making weight management simpler. Don't overlook the healthful fats found in foods like nuts, seeds, avocados, and olive oil. These fats are essential for brain development, joint function, and cardiovascular health.

Consuming them in moderation might have a positive impact on your overall health. Whole grains should also be a mainstay in your diet. Choose fiber-rich foods such as quinoa, brown rice, oats, and whole wheat bread to promote digestive health and energy generation.

Remain hydrated by drinking lots of water all day. Dehydration can increase age-related concerns including joint pain and weariness, so drink at least eight glasses of water every day.

In addition to a well-balanced diet, simple fitness workouts can help elders reduce weight and live a healthier lifestyle. Walking, swimming, tai chi, and gentle yoga are low-impact exercises that promote cardiovascular health, flexibility, and strength.

Begin with short sessions and progressively increase the intensity and duration as you gain stamina and confidence.

Healthy Snacking Strategies

Healthy snacking techniques are essential for preserving energy and achieving your fitness objectives. First, choose nutrient-dense foods such as fruits, vegetables, nuts, and whole grains. These include vital vitamins, minerals, and fiber, helping you stay full and satisfied.

Portion management is essential: Go for pre portioned snacks or single meals to avoid overeating. Go for pre portioned snacks or single meals to avoid overeating.

Include protein in your snacks to aid muscle regeneration and satiety. Greek yogurt, hard-boiled eggs, and a handful of almonds are also terrific options.

Mindful eating has an important function. Pay attention to your hunger signs and avoid munching out of boredom or stress. Instead, eat when you are truly hungry and quit when you are full.

To avoid making harmful decisions, plan beforehand. Preparing snacks ahead of time, such as chopping up vegetables or portioning out trail mix, will help you avoid the temptation of quick meals.

Hydration is sometimes underestimated yet critical for general health and satiety. Hunger can sometimes be confused with thirst. Drink water throughout the day, and consider hydrating snacks such as water-rich fruits and vegetables.

When it comes to senior fitness exercises for weight loss, choose low-impact sports that boost cardiovascular health and muscular strength. Walking, swimming, and cycling are terrific options. Chair exercises, resistance band workouts, and mild yoga can all assist in increasing flexibility and mobility without placing too much strain on joints.

Aim for at least 30 minutes of moderate-intensity activity most days of the week, gradually increasing the time and intensity as you go. Always listen to your body and talk with a doctor before beginning any new workout routine, especially if you have any underlying health issues.

Incorporating these healthy eating methods and fitness activities into your daily routine will help you lose weight and improve your overall health, keeping you feeling energized and powerful as you age. Remember that incremental, sustained adjustments result in long-term success.

Lifestyle Factors for Healthy Aging

Maintaining a healthy lifestyle as you become older is more important for your general well-being and lifespan. Several lifestyle variables contribute significantly to good aging.

First and foremost, prioritize regular physical activity. To increase cardiovascular health and endurance, perform a range of workouts, including aerobic activities such as walking, swimming, and cycling.

Include strength training routines to preserve muscle mass, bone density, and general strength. Pay strict attention to your nutrition. Choose a balanced diet high in fruits, vegetables, lean meats, whole grains, and healthy fats.

Limit your use of processed meals, sugary snacks, and high-sodium foods to promote good health and weight control. Adequate hydration is also required to sustain healthy body processes and general health.

Also, emphasize decent sleep. Aim for seven to nine hours of unbroken sleep every night to help your body relax, recoup, and renew. Create a consistent sleep schedule and a soothing nighttime ritual to improve sleep quality.

Also, manage stress well. Chronic stress can have a harmful influence on both physical and mental health, leading to a variety of age-related diseases. To increase calm and resilience, try stress-reduction strategies like mindfulness meditation, deep breathing exercises, and yoga.

Additionally, maintain social relationships. Strong social bonds can have a significant influence on general health and cognitive performance as you age.

Stay in touch with your friends, family, and community members by participating in frequent social events, volunteering, or joining groups and organizations.

When it comes to easy fitness exercises for seniors to lose weight, choose low-impact activities that are mild on the joints but efficient in burning calories.

Walking, water aerobics, tai chi, and moderate yoga are great alternatives for seniors who want to lose weight while increasing their general health.

These exercises may be changed to match a variety of fitness levels and physical abilities, making them appropriate for people of any age. Consistency is essential, so add these activities to your regimen multiple times each week for the best effects.

CONCLUSION

Easy fitness workouts designed specifically for seniors provide an efficient and accessible way to enhance weight reduction and general health. Walking, swimming, cycling, and chair exercises are examples of low-impact activities that seniors can do to improve their physical health and well-being.

These activities not only help with weight reduction, but they also bring various other advantages such as improved cardiovascular health, flexibility, muscular strength, and mood control.

The social component of group exercise programs or walking groups may develop a feeling of belonging and drive, enabling seniors to stick to a regular fitness regimen.

Importantly, safety and appropriate technique are crucial when performing these workouts. Seniors should check with a healthcare expert before starting any new exercise routine, especially if they have pre-existing health ailments or concerns.

Effective warm-up and cool-down routines, as well as hydration and body awareness, are critical strategies for avoiding injuries and having a great workout experience.

These workouts are simple and accessible, making them appropriate for seniors of various fitness levels and abilities. Easy fitness activities, whether done alone at home or as part of an organized program at a community center or gym, allow seniors to take charge of their health and well-being in a gentle yet effective way.

Easy fitness workouts for seniors might help them lose weight and enhance their health. Seniors who prioritize safety, accessibility, and enjoyment may gain the myriad physical, emotional, and social advantages of regular exercise.

With perseverance, support, and correct direction, seniors may adopt an active lifestyle and achieve their weight reduction objectives while improving their overall quality of life.

THANK YOU PAGE

Thank you for selecting this book. Your support is really appreciated. Similarly, I am grateful for the purchase of this book. Your input is valuable; please share your ideas in a review. It serves as a reference for future improvements. Enjoy reading and utilizing it!

30 Weeks Fitness planner to help track progress and improvements over time

Fitness Planner to Track progress

	EXERCISE	GOAL
MONDAY		
TUESDAY		
WEDNESDAY		
THURSDAY		
FRIDAY		
SATDAY		

Fitness Planner to Track progress

	EXERCISE	GOAL
MONDAY		
TUESDAY		
WEDNESDAY		
THURSDAY		
FRIDAY		
SATDAY		

Fitness Planner to Track progress

	EXERCISE	GOAL
MONDAY		
TUESDAY		
WEDNESDAY		
THURSDAY		
FRIDAY		
SATDAY		

Fitness Planner to Track progress

	EXERCISE	GOAL
MONDAY		
TUESDAY		
WEDNESDAY		
THURSDAY		
FRIDAY		
SATDAY		

Fitness Planner to Track progress

	EXERCISE	GOAL
MONDAY		
TUESDAY		
WEDNESDAY		
THURSDAY		
FRIDAY		
SATDAY		

Fitness Planner to Track progress

	EXERCISE	GOAL
MONDAY		
TUESDAY		
WEDNESDAY		
THURSDAY		
FRIDAY		
SATDAY		

Fitness Planner to Track progress

	EXERCISE	GOAL
MONDAY		
TUESDAY		
WEDNESDAY		
THURSDAY		
FRIDAY		
SATDAY		

Fitness Planner to Track progress

	EXERCISE	GOAL
MONDAY		
TUESDAY		
WEDNESDAY		
THURSDAY		
FRIDAY		
SATDAY		

Fitness Planner to Track progress

	EXERCISE	GOAL
MONDAY		
TUESDAY		
WEDNESDAY		
THURSDAY		
FRIDAY		
SATURDAY		

Fitness Planner to Track progress

	EXERCISE	GOAL
MONDAY		
TUESDAY		
WEDNESDAY		
THURSDAY		
FRIDAY		
SATDAY		

Fitness Planner to Track progress

	EXERCISE	GOAL
MONDAY		
TUESDAY		
WEDNESDAY		
THURSDAY		
FRIDAY		
SATDAY		

Fitness Planner to Track progress

	EXERCISE	GOAL
MONDAY		
TUESDAY		
WEDNESDAY		
THURSDAY		
FRIDAY		
SATDAY		

Fitness Planner to Track progress

	EXERCISE	GOAL
MONDAY		
TUESDAY		
WEDNESDAY		
THURSDAY		
FRIDAY		
SATDAY		

Fitness Planner to Track progress

	EXERCISE	GOAL
MONDAY		
TUESDAY		
WEDNESDAY		
THURSDAY		
FRIDAY		
SATDAY		

Fitness Planner to Track progress

	EXERCISE	GOAL
MONDAY		
TUESDAY		
WEDNESDAY		
THURSDAY		
FRIDAY		
SATDAY		

Fitness Planner to Track progress

	EXERCISE	GOAL
MONDAY		
TUESDAY		
WEDNESDAY		
THURSDAY		
FRIDAY		
SATDAY		

Fitness Planner to Track progress

	EXERCISE	GOAL
MONDAY		
TUESDAY		
WEDNESDAY		
THURSDAY		
FRIDAY		
SATDAY		

Fitness Planner to Track progress

	EXERCISE	GOAL
MONDAY		
TUESDAY		
WEDNESDAY		
THURSDAY		
FRIDAY		
SATDAY		

Fitness Planner to Track progress

	EXERCISE	GOAL
MONDAY		
TUESDAY		
WEDNESDAY		
THURSDAY		
FRIDAY		
SATDAY		

Fitness Planner to Track progress

	EXERCISE	GOAL
MONDAY		
TUESDAY		
WEDNESDAY		
THURSDAY		
FRIDAY		
SATDAY		

Fitness Planner to Track progress

	EXERCISE	GOAL
MONDAY		
TUESDAY		
WEDNESDAY		
THURSDAY		
FRIDAY		
SATDAY		

Fitness Planner to Track progress

	EXERCISE	GOAL
MONDAY		
TUESDAY		
WEDNESDAY		
THURSDAY		
FRIDAY		
SATDAY		

Fitness Planner to Track progress

	EXERCISE	GOAL
MONDAY		
TUESDAY		
WEDNESDAY		
THURSDAY		
FRIDAY		
SATDAY		

Fitness Planner to Track progress

	EXERCISE	GOAL
MONDAY		
TUESDAY		
WEDNESDAY		
THURSDAY		
FRIDAY		
SATDAY		

Fitness Planner to Track progress

	EXERCISE	GOAL
MONDAY		
TUESDAY		
WEDNESDAY		
THURSDAY		
FRIDAY		
SATDAY		

Fitness Planner to Track progress

	EXERCISE	GOAL
MONDAY		
TUESDAY		
WEDNESDAY		
THURSDAY		
FRIDAY		
SATDAY		

Fitness Planner to Track progress

	EXERCISE	GOAL
MONDAY		
TUESDAY		
WEDNESDAY		
THURSDAY		
FRIDAY		
SATDAY		

Fitness Planner to Track progress

	EXERCISE	GOAL
MONDAY		
TUESDAY		
WEDNESDAY		
THURSDAY		
FRIDAY		
SATDAY		

Fitness Planner to Track progress

	EXERCISE	GOAL
MONDAY		
TUESDAY		
WEDNESDAY		
THURSDAY		
FRIDAY		
SATDAY		

Fitness Planner to Track progress

	EXERCISE	GOAL
MONDAY		
TUESDAY		
WEDNESDAY		
THURSDAY		
FRIDAY		
SATDAY		

Fitness Planner to Track progress

	EXERCISE	GOAL
MONDAY		
TUESDAY		
WEDNESDAY		
THURSDAY		
FRIDAY		
SATDAY		

Fitness Planner to Track progress

	EXERCISE	GOAL
MONDAY		
TUESDAY		
WEDNESDAY		
THURSDAY		
FRIDAY		
SATDAY		

Printed in Dunstable, United Kingdom